LOW FODMAP DIET COOKBOOK

Delicious and Nutritious Recipes to Soothe Your Gut and Improve Digestion

Elise Norris

CONTENTS

INTRODUCTION

Definition and Explanation of the Low FODMAP Diet

The Low FODMAP Diet is a dietary approach designed to alleviate symptoms of certain gastrointestinal disorders, such as irritable bowel syndrome (IBS) and other functional gastrointestinal disorders. FODMAP stands for Fermentable Oligosaccharides, Disaccharides, Monosaccharides, and Polyols, which are a group of carbohydrates and sugar alcohols that can be poorly absorbed in the small intestine. When these substances are not adequately absorbed, they can ferment in the large intestine, leading to symptoms such as bloating, gas, abdominal pain, diarrhea, and constipation.

The diet was developed by researchers at Monash University in Australia, who identified specific foods that contain high levels of FODMAPs. The goal of the Low FODMAP Diet is to reduce the intake of these foods to minimize symptoms and improve the overall quality of life for individuals with gastrointestinal disorders.

To follow the Low FODMAP Diet, individuals need to avoid or limit the consumption of certain foods that are high in FODMAPs. These include:

1. **Oligosaccharides**: This group includes fructans and galacto-oligosaccharides (GOS), which are found in foods like wheat, rye, onions, garlic, legumes, and certain fruits and vegetables.

2. **Disaccharides**: Lactose, which is found in milk and dairy products, is the main disaccharide restricted in the diet.

3. **Monosaccharides**: Excess fructose, which is found in certain fruits, such as apples, pears, and honey, is limited in the Low FODMAP Diet.

4. **Polyols**: This group includes sugar alcohols like sorbitol, mannitol, xylitol, and maltitol, which are found in some fruits, artificial sweeteners, and sugar-free gums and candies.

By reducing the intake of high FODMAP foods, the diet aims to minimize the fermentation and subsequent production of gas in the gut, thereby alleviating symptoms associated with gastrointestinal disorders.

Purpose and Benefits of Following a Low FODMAP Diet

The primary purpose of following a Low FODMAP Diet is to manage and reduce the symptoms of gastrointestinal disorders, particularly IBS. The diet has been shown to be effective in improving symptoms such as bloating, gas, abdominal pain, diarrhea, and constipation in many individuals with these conditions.

Here are some key benefits of following a Low FODMAP Diet:

1. **Symptom Relief**: By eliminating or reducing high FODMAP foods, individuals can experience a significant reduction in the severity and frequency of their gastrointestinal symptoms. This can lead to improved quality of life and increased comfort.

2. **Individualized Approach**: The Low FODMAP Diet is not a one-size-fits-all approach. It involves a strict elimination phase followed by a structured reintroduction phase. This allows individuals to identify their specific trigger foods and customize their diet accordingly. It empowers them to make informed choices about their diet and manage their symptoms effectively.

3. **Scientifically Backed**: The Low FODMAP Diet has been extensively researched and is supported by a growing body of scientific evidence. Numerous studies have demonstrated its effectiveness in reducing symptoms and improving overall gut health.

4. **Nutritionally Balanced**: Although the diet restricts certain food groups, it is designed to

be nutritionally balanced. With proper guidance from a healthcare professional or registered dietitian, individuals can ensure they are meeting their nutritional needs while following the diet.

5. **Long-Term Management**: The Low FODMAP Diet can serve as a long-term management strategy for individuals with gastrointestinal disorders. While some may find relief by eliminating specific trigger foods permanently, others may be able to reintroduce some high FODMAP foods in moderation without triggering symptoms.

It's important to note that the Low FODMAP Diet is not intended as a long-term solution for everyone. It should be followed under the guidance of a healthcare professional or registered dietitian who can provide appropriate advice and support.

Target Audience for the eBook

The target audience for the eBook on the Low FODMAP Diet can include individuals who are seeking relief from symptoms associated with gastrointestinal disorders, particularly IBS. This can include people of varying ages and backgrounds who have been diagnosed with these conditions or suspect they may have them.

The eBook can also be valuable for healthcare

professionals, including doctors, gastroenterologists, and dietitians, who work with patients suffering from gastrointestinal disorders. It can serve as a comprehensive resource to educate their patients about the Low FODMAP Diet, its principles, and how to effectively implement it.

Additionally, individuals who are interested in learning about gut health, nutrition, and dietary strategies for managing digestive symptoms can find the eBook beneficial. It can provide them with a clear understanding of the Low FODMAP Diet, enabling them to make informed decisions about their own health and explore potential solutions to their symptoms.

The eBook should be written in a clear and accessible manner, providing practical tips, meal plans, recipes, and strategies for successfully implementing the Low FODMAP Diet. It should aim to empower the readers, educate them about the diet's potential benefits, and guide them through the process of implementing it effectively.

Overall, the eBook can be a valuable resource for individuals with gastrointestinal disorders, healthcare professionals, and anyone interested in improving gut health and managing digestive symptoms through dietary interventions.

CHAPTER ONE

Understanding FODMAPs

Explanation of FODMAPs and their role in digestive health

FODMAPs, which stands for Fermentable Oligosaccharides, Disaccharides, Monosaccharides, and Polyols, are a group of carbohydrates and sugar alcohols that are known to cause digestive symptoms in certain individuals. These substances are poorly absorbed in the small intestine and can ferment in the colon, leading to symptoms such as bloating, gas, abdominal pain, and changes in bowel movements.

The role of FODMAPs in digestive health revolves around their ability to draw water into the intestines and produce gas when fermented by bacteria. For people with sensitive digestive systems, FODMAPs can be difficult to digest and absorb properly. This can result in an imbalance in the gut microbiota, leading to discomfort and symptoms associated with irritable bowel syndrome (IBS) and other gastrointestinal disorders.

Common foods high in FODMAPs

FODMAPs are present in a wide range of foods. Here are some examples of common foods that are high in FODMAPs:

1. **Oligosaccharides**: Foods high in oligosaccharides include wheat, rye, barley, onions, garlic, chickpeas, lentils, and legumes. These carbohydrates are made up of short chains of sugar molecules that are not easily broken down during digestion.

2. **Disaccharides**: Lactose, a disaccharide found in milk and dairy products, is a common FODMAP. People who are lactose intolerant have difficulty digesting lactose due to a deficiency of the enzyme lactase.

3. **Monosaccharides**: Fructose, a monosaccharide found in fruits, honey, and some sweeteners, can be a source of FODMAPs. High levels of fructose can overwhelm the small intestine's capacity to absorb it, leading to malabsorption and symptoms.

4. **Polyols**: Polyols, also known as sugar alcohols,

are found in certain fruits (such as apples, pears, and stone fruits), as well as in some artificial sweeteners like xylitol, sorbitol, and mannitol. These compounds are poorly absorbed and can have a laxative effect.

It's important to note that not all individuals are equally sensitive to FODMAPs, and the amount of FODMAPs that triggers symptoms can vary from person to person. Additionally, some foods may contain a mixture of different types of FODMAPs, making it challenging to pinpoint specific triggers.

How FODMAPs can trigger digestive symptoms

FODMAPs can trigger digestive symptoms through several mechanisms. When FODMAPs are poorly absorbed in the small intestine, they continue their journey to the colon, where they become food for the bacteria residing there. The fermentation process produces gases, such as hydrogen and methane, which can cause bloating, distension, and flatulence.

Furthermore, FODMAPs have an osmotic effect, meaning they draw water into the intestines. This increased fluid volume can lead to diarrhea and loose stools in individuals with FODMAP sensitivity.

In addition to the physical effects, FODMAPs can also act as irritants to the gut lining. In individuals with a compromised gut barrier, these substances may trigger inflammation and further contribute to digestive symptoms.

It's worth noting that the effects of FODMAPs are highly individualized. Some people may be able to tolerate certain FODMAP-containing foods in small amounts without experiencing symptoms, while others may need to strictly avoid them.

CHAPTER TWO

Benefits of a Low FODMAP Diet

Reduction of Digestive Symptoms

Digestive symptoms such as bloating, gas, constipation, and diarrhea can significantly impact a person's quality of life. However, there are various approaches to reduce these symptoms and promote better digestive health. Here are some strategies that can help alleviate digestive discomfort:

1. **Dietary Modifications:** Making changes to your diet can play a crucial role in reducing digestive symptoms. One approach is to identify and avoid foods that trigger discomfort. Common culprits include spicy foods, fatty foods, caffeine, alcohol, and certain types of carbohydrates known as FODMAPs. Adopting a low-FODMAP diet may provide relief for individuals with conditions like irritable bowel syndrome (IBS).

2. **Increased Fiber Intake:** Consuming an adequate amount of dietary fiber can help regulate bowel movements and relieve constipation. Whole grains, fruits, vegetables, legumes, and nuts are excellent sources of fiber. Gradually increasing fiber intake and ensuring adequate hydration can aid in reducing digestive issues.

3. **Probiotics:** Probiotics are beneficial bacteria that can promote a healthy gut. They are available as supplements or can be found naturally in fermented foods like yogurt, kefir, sauerkraut, and kimchi. Probiotics have been shown to alleviate symptoms of bloating, gas, and diarrhea, particularly in individuals with conditions such as IBS.

4. **Stress Reduction:** High levels of stress can exacerbate digestive symptoms. Practicing stress management techniques like meditation, deep breathing exercises, yoga, or engaging in hobbies and activities that promote relaxation can have a positive impact on gut health. Additionally, regular exercise is known to reduce stress and improve overall well-being.

5. **Hydration:** Staying adequately hydrated is essential for maintaining healthy digestion. Drinking enough water helps soften stools, prevent constipation, and facilitate the movement of food through the digestive system. Aim to drink at least eight glasses of water per day and increase fluid intake during hot weather or physical activity.

6. **Chewing and Eating Habits:** Proper chewing and

mindful eating can aid digestion. Chewing food thoroughly helps break it down into smaller particles, making it easier for the digestive system to process. Eating slowly and avoiding large meals can also prevent overeating and reduce the likelihood of digestive discomfort.

It's important to note that while these strategies may help alleviate digestive symptoms, it's always advisable to consult with a healthcare professional, particularly if the symptoms persist or worsen.

Improved Gut Health

Maintaining a healthy gut is vital for overall well-being as it plays a significant role in digestion, nutrient absorption, immune function, and even mental health. Several factors contribute to a healthy gut, and adopting certain practices can promote its optimal functioning. Here are some ways to improve gut health:

1. **Balanced Diet:** Consuming a balanced diet rich in diverse nutrients is essential for supporting gut health. Include a variety of fruits, vegetables, whole grains, lean proteins, and healthy fats in your meals. This diverse range of nutrients provides essential building blocks for the gut microbiota, the collection of bacteria residing in the digestive system.

2. **Fiber-Rich Foods:** As mentioned earlier, fiber is

crucial for maintaining a healthy gut. It acts as a prebiotic, serving as fuel for the beneficial bacteria in the gut. Incorporate plenty of fiber-rich foods such as whole grains, legumes, fruits, and vegetables into your diet to support a thriving gut microbiome.

3. **Probiotics and Fermented Foods:** Probiotics are live bacteria that offer health benefits when consumed. They can be taken as supplements or obtained from fermented foods like yogurt, kefir, sauerkraut, and kombucha. Probiotics help maintain a diverse and balanced gut microbiota, contributing to better digestive health.

4. **Avoidance of Antibiotic Overuse:** While antibiotics are essential for fighting bacterial infections, their overuse can disrupt the balance of gut bacteria. If prescribed antibiotics, ensure you follow the recommended course and consider taking probiotics during and after the treatment to support the restoration of a healthy gut microbiome.

5. **Adequate Sleep:** Sufficient and restful sleep is crucial for maintaining a healthy gut. Sleep deprivation can disrupt the gut microbiota and increase the risk of gastrointestinal issues. Aim for 7-9 hours of quality sleep per night to support optimal gut health.

6. **Regular Exercise:** Engaging in regular physical activity has been shown to positively influence gut health. Exercise promotes better digestion, enhances blood flow to the intestines, and stimulates the gut muscles. Aim for at least 150

minutes of moderate-intensity exercise per week to reap the benefits for your gut and overall health.

Potential Relief for Individuals with Irritable Bowel Syndrome (IBS)

Irritable bowel syndrome (IBS) is a common gastrointestinal disorder characterized by recurring abdominal pain, bloating, changes in bowel habits, and other digestive symptoms. While there is no cure for IBS, certain interventions can help manage and alleviate its symptoms. Here are some potential relief strategies for individuals with IBS:

1. **Low-FODMAP Diet:** The low-FODMAP diet is an evidence-based approach that involves restricting fermentable carbohydrates that may trigger IBS symptoms. FODMAPs are found in a variety of foods such as wheat, onions, garlic, certain fruits, and artificial sweeteners. Working with a registered dietitian can help determine which specific foods trigger symptoms and create an individualized low-FODMAP plan.

2. **Stress Management:** Stress can worsen IBS symptoms, so finding effective stress management techniques is crucial. Regular exercise, meditation, deep breathing exercises, and therapy (such as cognitive-behavioral therapy) can help individuals cope with stress and

reduce the impact on their digestive system.

3. **Medication:** In some cases, healthcare providers may prescribe medication to manage specific symptoms of IBS. For instance, antispasmodic medications can help reduce abdominal pain and cramping. Additionally, laxatives or anti-diarrheal agents may be recommended to address constipation or diarrhea, respectively. It's important to consult with a healthcare professional to determine the most appropriate medication for individual needs.

4. **Probiotics:** Probiotics, as mentioned earlier, can be beneficial for individuals with IBS. They help modulate gut bacteria and may provide relief for symptoms such as bloating, gas, and abdominal pain. However, the effectiveness of probiotics may vary depending on the specific strains and individuals, so it's advisable to consult with a healthcare professional before starting any supplementation.

5. **Identifying Trigger Foods:** Keeping a food diary and tracking symptoms can help identify specific trigger foods that worsen IBS symptoms. By eliminating or reducing the consumption of these trigger foods, individuals may experience relief from their digestive discomfort.

6. **Lifestyle Modifications:** Implementing healthy lifestyle habits can contribute to overall well-being and help manage IBS symptoms. This includes regular physical activity, adequate sleep, maintaining a balanced diet, and avoiding smoking and excessive alcohol consumption.

While these strategies can provide relief for individuals with IBS, it's essential to work closely with healthcare professionals, such as gastroenterologists and dietitians, to create a personalized management plan that suits individual needs.

CHAPTER THREE

Getting Started with a Low FODMAP Diet

Consulting with a healthcare professional or registered dietitian

When it comes to managing your health and making informed decisions about your diet, consulting with a healthcare professional or registered dietitian is an essential step. These experts have the knowledge and experience to guide you on your journey towards better health and well-being. Whether you're dealing with a specific health condition, seeking weight loss advice, or simply looking to optimize your diet, a consultation with a healthcare professional or registered dietitian can provide invaluable support. In this article, we'll explore the benefits of consulting with these professionals and highlight the key aspects of the process.

The Benefits of Consulting with a Healthcare Professional or Registered Dietitian

1. **Expertise and Knowledge:** Healthcare professionals and registered dietitians undergo extensive education and training in their respective fields. They stay up-to-date with the latest research and guidelines, ensuring that you receive accurate and evidence-based information. Their expertise enables them to provide personalized advice tailored to your specific needs and goals.

2. **Health Assessment:** During a consultation, a healthcare professional or registered dietitian will conduct a thorough assessment of your health status, medical history, lifestyle, and dietary habits. This assessment allows them to understand your unique circumstances and develop an individualized plan that addresses your specific concerns.

3. **Specialized Guidance:** If you have a particular health condition or dietary requirement, consulting with a healthcare professional or registered dietitian is especially important. These professionals can provide specialized guidance for conditions such as diabetes, heart disease, food allergies, gastrointestinal disorders, and more. They can help you navigate complex dietary restrictions and create a balanced meal plan that meets your nutritional needs.

4. **Behavioral Change Support:** Changing dietary habits and adopting a healthier lifestyle can

be challenging. A healthcare professional or registered dietitian can offer valuable support and motivation throughout your journey. They can assist you in setting realistic goals, developing strategies to overcome barriers, and providing ongoing accountability to help you stay on track.

The Process of Consulting with a Healthcare Professional or Registered Dietitian

1. **Finding a Professional:** Start by finding a reputable healthcare professional or registered dietitian in your area. You can ask for recommendations from your primary care physician, friends, or family members. Additionally, professional organizations and online directories can help you locate qualified practitioners.

2. **Scheduling an Appointment:** Once you have identified a potential professional, contact their office to schedule an appointment. Depending on the availability and urgency, you may need to book the appointment in advance. Be prepared to provide basic information about your health, medical history, and reason for seeking consultation.

3. **Preparing for the Consultation:** Before the appointment, gather any relevant medical reports, test results, or previous diet records that may be useful for the healthcare professional or registered dietitian to review. It can also be helpful to write down any questions or concerns you have, ensuring that you make the most of

your consultation.

4. **The Consultation:** During the consultation, the healthcare professional or registered dietitian will ask you detailed questions about your health, lifestyle, dietary habits, and goals. They may also conduct measurements such as body weight, height, and body composition analysis. This information helps them tailor their advice specifically to you.

5. **Creating an Action Plan:** Based on the information gathered, the healthcare professional or registered dietitian will develop an action plan that outlines specific dietary and lifestyle recommendations. This plan may include meal suggestions, portion control guidance, tips for managing cravings, and strategies for overcoming potential obstacles. They may also provide educational resources to enhance your understanding of nutrition and health.

6. **Follow-up Appointments:** Depending on your needs and goals, follow-up appointments may be scheduled to monitor your progress, make adjustments to the action plan, and address any additional questions or concerns. Follow-up appointments provide an opportunity to evaluate your response to the recommendations and ensure continued support on your health journey.

Consulting with a healthcare professional or registered dietitian empowers you to make informed decisions about your health and well-being. Their expertise, guidance, and ongoing support can significantly improve your chances of achieving your health goals and maintaining a balanced lifestyle. Remember, your health is a valuable investment, and seeking professional advice is a proactive step towards taking care of yourself.

Step-by-Step Guide to Eliminating High FODMAP Foods

If you've been experiencing digestive issues such as bloating, gas, or abdominal pain, you may have heard about the low FODMAP diet. FODMAPs (fermentable oligosaccharides, disaccharides, monosaccharides, and polyols) are a group of carbohydrates that can be difficult for some people to digest. Eliminating high FODMAP foods from your diet may help alleviate symptoms and improve your digestive health. In this step-by-step guide, we'll walk you through the process of eliminating high FODMAP foods.

Step 1: Educate Yourself about FODMAPs

1. **Understand the Basics:** Familiarize yourself with the concept of FODMAPs and the role they play in gastrointestinal symptoms. Learn about the different types of FODMAPs, such as lactose, fructose, and sorbitol, and the foods that contain them.

2. **Consult a Professional:** While it's possible to educate yourself using reputable online resources, consulting with a healthcare professional or registered dietitian who specializes in the low FODMAP diet is highly recommended. They can provide personalized guidance and ensure that you're following the diet correctly.

Step 2: Identify High FODMAP Foods

1. **Review FODMAP Food Lists:** Access reliable resources that provide comprehensive lists of high FODMAP foods. These lists categorize foods according to their FODMAP content, making it easier for you to identify which ones to avoid.

2. **Be Mindful of Serving Sizes:** Keep in mind that the FODMAP content of certain foods may vary depending on the portion size. Take note of recommended serving sizes to ensure you're accurately assessing your intake.

Step 3: Eliminate High FODMAP Foods from Your Diet

1. **Go Cold Turkey or Gradually:** Decide whether you prefer to eliminate high FODMAP foods all at once or gradually phase them out. Some individuals find it easier to make a clean break, while others may benefit from a more gradual approach.

2. **Plan Your Meals:** Explore low FODMAP recipe sources and meal ideas to ensure you have a variety of options available. Consider working with a registered dietitian to create a meal

plan that meets your nutritional needs and preferences.

Step 4: Monitor Your Symptoms

1. **Keep a Food Diary:** Document your meals and note any changes in your symptoms. This will help you identify potential trigger foods and track your progress over time.

2. **Reintroduction Phase:** After a period of strict FODMAP elimination, you'll enter the reintroduction phase. Under the guidance of a healthcare professional or registered dietitian, you'll systematically reintroduce FODMAPs to identify which specific carbohydrates may be triggering your symptoms.

Step 5: Personalize Your Diet

1. **Reintroduce Tolerated FODMAPs:** Once you've identified your personal FODMAP triggers, you can reintroduce and enjoy FODMAP-containing foods that you tolerate well. This will help expand your diet and maintain a balanced nutritional intake

2. **Modify Recipes:** Adapt your favorite recipes to make them low in FODMAPs. Look for suitable ingredient substitutions and experiment with different flavors and spices to enhance the taste of your meals.

3. **Seek Professional Guidance:** As you personalize your diet, it's important to consult with a healthcare professional or registered dietitian. They can provide ongoing support, help you

navigate food choices, and ensure that you maintain a balanced and nutritionally adequate diet.

Step 6: Maintain a Balanced Diet

1. **Focus on Nutrient-Rich Foods:** While eliminating high FODMAP foods, it's crucial to ensure that you're still consuming a wide range of nutrients. Prioritize nutrient-dense foods such as lean proteins, fruits, vegetables, whole grains, and healthy fats.

2. **Consider Supplementation:** If you're eliminating a large number of high FODMAP foods from your diet, you may want to discuss potential nutrient gaps with your healthcare professional or registered dietitian. They can guide you on appropriate supplementation if needed.

Step 7: Seek Support and Adaptation

1. **Find Supportive Communities:** Connecting with others who are following a low FODMAP diet can provide encouragement, recipe ideas, and emotional support. Look for online communities, forums, or support groups where you can share experiences and learn from others.

2. **Be Flexible and Adapt:** The low FODMAP diet is not meant to be a lifelong restriction. Once you've identified your triggers, you can reintroduce tolerated FODMAPs and enjoy a varied diet. Be open to adjusting your eating plan as needed and listen to your body's cues.

Identifying Potential Sources of Hidden FODMAPs

While eliminating high FODMAP foods is essential for managing symptoms, it's equally important to be aware of potential sources of hidden FODMAPs. These are foods or ingredients that may contain FODMAPs but are not immediately obvious. By identifying and avoiding these hidden sources, you can maintain better control over your FODMAP intake. Here are some key points to consider:

1. **Read Food Labels:** When grocery shopping, carefully read food labels to check for ingredients that may contain FODMAPs. Common culprits include wheat, high fructose corn syrup, onion or garlic powder, and certain artificial sweeteners like sorbitol or mannitol.

2. **Beware of Processed Foods:** Processed foods, such as ready-made meals, sauces, dressings, and snacks, often contain hidden FODMAPs. These can include added sugars, flavorings, or preservatives that may trigger symptoms. Opt for homemade or low FODMAP certified alternatives whenever possible.

3. **Watch Out for Cross-Contamination:** In restaurants or shared kitchen environments, cross-contamination can occur when utensils or cooking surfaces are used for both high FODMAP and low FODMAP foods. This can introduce FODMAPs into otherwise safe dishes. Communicate your dietary needs clearly and ask

about food preparation methods to minimize the risk.

4. **Consider Medications and Supplements:** Some medications and dietary supplements may contain FODMAP ingredients or additives. Discuss your medication and supplement regimen with your healthcare professional or registered dietitian to ensure they are compatible with your low FODMAP diet.

5. **Stay Informed and Updated:** Keep yourself informed about new research, food labeling regulations, and low FODMAP certified products. Stay connected with healthcare professionals, registered dietitians, and reputable online resources to stay up-to-date on the latest information.

By being diligent in reading labels, choosing whole foods, and staying informed, you can minimize your exposure to hidden sources of FODMAPs and maintain better control over your symptoms.

Consulting with a healthcare professional or registered dietitian, following a step-by-step guide to eliminating high FODMAP foods, and being aware of potential hidden sources of FODMAPs are crucial steps in managing digestive symptoms and optimizing your overall well-being. Remember, everyone's experience with FODMAPs is unique, so it's essential to work with a professional to develop an individualized approach that suits your specific needs and health goals.

CHAPTER FOUR

Low FODMAP Food List

Detailed list of low FODMAP foods across different food groups

Following a low FODMAP (Fermentable Oligosaccharides, Disaccharides, Monosaccharides, and Polyols) diet can be challenging, but it is manageable with the right information and food choices. This diet aims to reduce the intake of certain carbohydrates that can trigger digestive symptoms in individuals with irritable bowel syndrome (IBS) or other digestive disorders. Here is a detailed list of low FODMAP foods across different food groups:

Fruits

1. **Citrus fruits**: Oranges, lemons, limes, and grapefruits are generally low in FODMAPs and can be enjoyed in moderation.

2. **Berries**: Strawberries, blueberries, raspberries, and blackberries are low FODMAP fruits that can be added to your diet.

3. **Bananas**: Ripe bananas are a good choice as they are low in FODMAPs, while unripe ones are high in resistant starch.

4. **Grapes**: Both red and green grapes are low FODMAP options.

5. **Kiwi**: Kiwi is a delicious low FODMAP fruit rich in vitamin C and fiber.

6. **Pineapple**: Enjoy fresh pineapple in moderate amounts.

7. **Cantaloupe**: A low FODMAP melon that can be included in your diet.

Vegetables

1. **Leafy greens**: Spinach, kale, lettuce, and other leafy greens are typically low in FODMAPs and provide essential nutrients.

2. **Carrots**: Carrots are a versatile low FODMAP vegetable that can be used in various dishes.

3. **Bell peppers**: Both red and green bell peppers are low FODMAP options.

4. **Zucchini**: Zucchini is a low FODMAP vegetable that can be spiralized or used in stir-fries.

5. **Tomatoes**: Ripe tomatoes are considered low FODMAP, while cherry tomatoes should be consumed in moderation.

6. **Cucumbers**: Cucumbers are refreshing and low in FODMAPs.

7. **Potatoes**: Regular potatoes and sweet potatoes are low FODMAP choices, but watch out for high FODMAP toppings or seasonings.

Proteins

1. **Meat**: Most unprocessed meats, such as chicken, turkey, beef, and pork, are low in FODMAPs.

2. **Fish**: Fish like salmon, tuna, cod, and haddock are low FODMAP protein sources.

3. **Eggs**: Eggs are a versatile and low FODMAP protein option.

4. **Tofu**: Firm tofu is a suitable low FODMAP choice for vegetarians and vegans.

5. **Quinoa**: Quinoa is a pseudo-grain that is low in FODMAPs and can be used as a protein source.

Grains and Cereals

1. **Rice**: White, brown, and basmati rice are all low FODMAP options.

2. **Oats**: Gluten-free oats are low in FODMAPs and can be enjoyed in moderation.

3. **Corn**: Cornmeal, cornflour, and corn tortillas are low FODMAP choices.

4. **Gluten-free bread**: Look for gluten-free bread made with low FODMAP ingredients like rice flour or sourdough spelt bread.

5. **Buckwheat**: Buckwheat is a low FODMAP grain alternative that can be used in pancakes, porridge, or as a side dish.

Dairy Alternatives

1. **Lactose-free milk**: Lactose-free milk is a suitable alternative for those following a low FODMAP diet.

2. **Almond milk**: Unsweetened almond milk is low in FODMAPs and can be used as a dairy substitute.

3. **Coconut milk**: Coconut milk is a creamy and low FODMAP option for cooking and baking.

4. **Hard cheeses**: Some hard cheeses, like cheddar, Swiss, and Parmesan, are low in lactose and FODMAPs.

Remember, portion sizes and individual tolerances may vary, so it's essential to work with a registered dietitian or healthcare professional to create a personalized low FODMAP meal plan that suits your needs.

7 Days Sample meal plans

Creating a 7-day sample meal plan while following a low FODMAP diet can provide structure and variety to your eating routine. Here's a sample meal plan to help you get started:

Day 1

- **Breakfast**: Omelette with spinach, bell peppers, and lactose-free cheese.
- **Lunch**: Grilled chicken salad with mixed greens, cherry tomatoes, cucumbers, and balsamic

vinaigrette.

- **Snack**: A handful of almonds and a small bunch of grapes.
- **Dinner**: Baked salmon with lemon, served with quinoa and steamed carrots.
- **Dessert**: A small bowl of strawberries.

Day 2

- **Breakfast**: Gluten-free oatmeal topped with sliced bananas and a sprinkle of cinnamon.
- **Lunch**: Quinoa salad with grilled tofu, mixed vegetables, and a low FODMAP dressing.
- **Snack**: Carrot sticks with lactose-free yogurt dip.
- **Dinner**: Beef stir-fry with zucchini, bell peppers, and gluten-free soy sauce, served over rice.
- **Dessert**: A small slice of lactose-free cheesecake.

Day 3

- **Breakfast**: Scrambled eggs with spinach, tomatoes, and a side of gluten-free toast.
- **Lunch**: Turkey lettuce wraps with cucumber, bell peppers, and a low FODMAP sauce.
- **Snack**: Rice cakes with natural peanut butter.
- **Dinner**: Grilled chicken breast with roasted potatoes and a side of steamed broccoli.
- **Dessert**: A small portion of lactose-free vanilla ice cream.

Day 4

- **Breakfast**: Rice cakes with almond butter and sliced kiwi.
- **Lunch**: Spinach salad with grilled shrimp, cherry

tomatoes, and a low FODMAP dressing.

- **Snack**: A handful of mixed nuts.
- **Dinner**: Pork tenderloin with roasted sweet potatoes and sautéed zucchini.
- **Dessert**: Fresh pineapple chunks.

Day 5

- **Breakfast**: Smoothie made with lactose-free yogurt, strawberries, and a scoop of protein powder.
- **Lunch**: Chicken and vegetable soup made with low FODMAP ingredients.
- **Snack**: Rice crackers with lactose-free cream cheese.
- **Dinner**: Baked cod with lemon and herbs, served with quinoa and steamed asparagus.
- **Dessert**: A small piece of dark chocolate.

Day 6

- **Breakfast**: Gluten-free pancakes with maple syrup and blueberries.
- **Lunch**: Tuna salad with mixed greens, cucumbers, and a low FODMAP dressing.
- **Snack**: Sliced bell peppers with hummus.
- **Dinner**: Grilled steak with roasted potatoes and a side of sautéed spinach.
- **Dessert**: A small bowl of mixed berries.

Day 7

- **Breakfast**: Quinoa porridge with almond milk, topped with sliced bananas and a drizzle of maple syrup.

- **Lunch**: Grilled chicken wrap with lettuce, tomatoes, and lactose-free mayo, served with a side of carrot sticks.
- **Snack**: Rice cakes with a spread of sunflower seed butter.
- **Dinner**: Baked tofu with stir-fried bok choy, bell peppers, and gluten-free soy sauce, served over rice.
- **Dessert**: A small serving of lactose-free coconut milk yogurt.

Feel free to modify these sample meal plans based on your individual preferences and dietary needs. Remember to check ingredient labels carefully, as some packaged foods may contain hidden sources of FODMAPs. It's always a good idea to consult with a registered dietitian or healthcare professional for personalized guidance and support.

Recipes

Grilled Chicken Breast with Steamed Carrots and a Side Salad

Description: This healthy and flavorful meal features tender grilled chicken breast accompanied by steamed carrots and a refreshing side salad. The grilled chicken is juicy and seasoned to perfection, while the steamed carrots provide a touch of natural sweetness. The side salad adds a fresh and crisp element to the dish, making it a well-rounded and satisfying meal.

Ingredients:

- 2 chicken breasts
- 4 medium carrots
- Mixed salad greens
- Cherry tomatoes
- Cucumber
- Red onion
- Balsamic vinaigrette dressing

Instructions:

1. Preheat the grill to medium-high heat.
2. Season the chicken breasts with salt, pepper, and your preferred seasonings.
3. Grill the chicken breasts for about 6-8 minutes per side or until cooked through. Let them rest for a few minutes before slicing.
4. While the chicken is grilling, peel and slice the carrots into thin rounds. Steam them until tender.
5. In a large bowl, combine the mixed salad greens, cherry tomatoes (halved), sliced cucumber, and thinly sliced red onion.
6. Drizzle the salad with balsamic vinaigrette dressing and toss gently to coat.

7. Serve the grilled chicken slices alongside the steamed carrots and the side salad.

Nutritional Information:

- Calories: 350-400 per serving
- Protein: 30-40g
- Carbohydrates: 20-30g
- Fat: 10-15g
- Fiber: 5-8g

Baked Salmon with Roasted Zucchini and Quinoa

Description: This delightful dish showcases succulent baked salmon paired with flavorful roasted zucchini and a bed of nutty quinoa. The salmon is seasoned with herbs and spices, resulting in a perfectly cooked, tender, and flaky texture. The roasted zucchini adds a hint of smokiness, while the quinoa provides a wholesome and protein-packed base for the dish.

Ingredients:

- 2 salmon fillets
- 2 medium zucchini
- 1 cup quinoa
- Olive oil
- Garlic powder
- Dried dill
- Salt and pepper

Instructions:

1. Preheat the oven to 400°F (200°C).

2. Place the salmon fillets on a baking sheet lined with parchment paper. Drizzle with olive oil and season with garlic powder, dried dill, salt, and pepper.

3. Cut the zucchini into bite-sized pieces and place them on another baking sheet. Drizzle with olive oil and season with salt and pepper.

4. Bake the salmon and zucchini in the preheated oven for about 15-20 minutes or until the salmon is cooked through and flakes easily with a fork.

5. While the salmon and zucchini are baking, cook the quinoa according to package instructions.

6. Once cooked, fluff the quinoa with a fork and season with salt and pepper to taste.

7. Serve the baked salmon on a bed of quinoa, with the roasted zucchini on the side.

Nutritional Information:

- Calories: 400-450 per serving
- Protein: 30-35g
- Carbohydrates: 30-35g
- Fat: 15-20g
- Fiber: 5-7g

Stir-Fried Tofu with Bell Peppers, Broccoli, and Brown Rice

Description: This flavorful stir-fried tofu dish combines the goodness of protein-rich tofu with vibrant bell peppers and nutritious broccoli. Served over a bed of nutty brown rice, this meal is both satisfying and wholesome. The combination of colors, textures, and flavors makes it a delightful option for a vegetarian or vegan dinner.

Ingredients:

- 1 block of firm tofu
- 1 red bell pepper
- 1 yellow bell pepper
- 1 green bell pepper
- 1 head of broccoli
- 2 cups cooked brown rice
- Soy sauce
- Sesame oil
- Garlic powder
- Ginger powder
- Red pepper flakes (optional)

Instructions:

1. Drain and press the tofu to remove excess moisture. Cut the tofu into cubes.

2. Cut the bell peppers into strips and the broccoli into florets.

3. Heat sesame oil in a large pan or wok over medium-high heat.

4. Add the tofu cubes to the pan and cook until lightly browned on all sides. Remove from the pan and set aside.

5. In the same pan, add a little more sesame oil if needed. Stir-fry the bell peppers and broccoli until they are tender-crisp.

6. Add the cooked tofu back to the pan.

7. Season with soy sauce, garlic powder, ginger powder, and red pepper flakes (if desired). Toss everything together to coat evenly.

8. Serve the stir-fried tofu, bell peppers, and broccoli over a bed of cooked brown rice.

Nutritional Information:

- Calories: 400-450 per serving
- Protein: 20-25g
- Carbohydrates: 50-60g
- Fat: 10-15g
- Fiber: 8-10g

Shrimp and Vegetable Skewers served with a Side of Jasmine Rice

Description: This delightful meal features succulent

shrimp and colorful vegetables threaded onto skewers, grilled to perfection. Served alongside fragrant jasmine rice, this dish is bursting with flavors and textures. The juicy shrimp and charred vegetables create a mouthwatering combination, making it a satisfying and healthy option for any seafood lover.

Ingredients:

- 1 pound shrimp, peeled and deveined
- 1 red bell pepper
- 1 green bell pepper
- 1 yellow bell pepper
- 1 red onion
- 1 zucchini
- Wooden or metal skewers
- 2 cups cooked jasmine rice
- Olive oil
- Garlic powder
- Paprika
- Salt and pepper

Instructions:

1. If using wooden skewers, soak them in water for about 30 minutes to prevent burning during grilling.
2. Preheat the grill to medium-high heat.
3. Cut the bell peppers, red onion, and zucchini into

bite-sized pieces.

4. Thread the shrimp, bell peppers, red onion, and zucchini onto the skewers, alternating between ingredients.

5. Drizzle the skewers with olive oil and season with garlic powder, paprika, salt, and pepper.

6. Grill the skewers for about 3-4 minutes per side or until the shrimp is cooked through and the vegetables are slightly charred.

7. While the skewers are grilling, cook the jasmine rice according to package instructions.

8. Serve the shrimp and vegetable skewers alongside a portion of fragrant jasmine rice.

Nutritional Information:

- Calories: 350-400 per serving
- Protein: 25-30g
- Carbohydrates: 40-45g
- Fat: 5-8g
- Fiber: 3-5g

Quinoa Salad with Cucumber, Cherry Tomatoes, and Feta Cheese

Description: This refreshing and nutritious salad combines fluffy quinoa with crisp cucumber, juicy cherry tomatoes, and tangy feta cheese. It's a light yet satisfying meal that can be enjoyed as a standalone dish or as a side.

The combination of flavors and textures, along with the protein-rich quinoa, makes this salad a well-balanced and delicious option.

Ingredients:

- 1 cup cooked quinoa
- 1 English cucumber
- 1 cup cherry tomatoes, halved
- ½ cup crumbled feta cheese
- Fresh parsley, chopped
- Lemon juice
- Olive oil
- Salt and pepper

Instructions:

1. In a large bowl, combine the cooked quinoa, sliced cucumber, halved cherry tomatoes, crumbled feta cheese, and chopped fresh parsley.
2. Drizzle the salad with lemon juice and olive oil.
3. Season with salt and pepper to taste.
4. Toss gently to combine all the ingredients and ensure even dressing distribution.
5. Let the salad sit for a few minutes to allow the flavors to meld together.
6. Serve the quinoa salad as a light and refreshing meal on its own or as a side dish.

Nutritional Information:

- Calories: 300-350 per serving
- Protein: 10-12g
- Carbohydrates: 40-45g
- Fat: 10-12g
- Fiber: 6-8g

Grilled Steak with Sautéed Spinach and Mashed Sweet Potatoes

Description: Indulge in a hearty and satisfying meal with juicy grilled steak, flavorful sautéed spinach, and creamy mashed sweet potatoes. The grilled steak is seasoned to perfection, while the sautéed spinach adds a burst of vibrant green goodness. Paired with creamy mashed sweet potatoes, this dish offers a harmonious blend of flavors and textures that will leave you feeling satisfied and nourished.

Ingredients:

- 2 steaks (your preferred cut)
- 4 cups fresh spinach leaves
- 2 large sweet potatoes
- Butter or ghee
- Milk (dairy or plant-based)
- Garlic powder
- Salt and pepper

Instructions:

1. Preheat the grill to medium-high heat.

2. Season the steaks with salt, pepper, and garlic powder.

3. Grill the steaks for about 4-6 minutes per side, depending on your preferred level of doneness. Allow them to rest for a few minutes before slicing.

4. While the steaks are grilling, wash the spinach leaves and set them aside.

5. Peel and chop the sweet potatoes into chunks.

6. Boil the sweet potato chunks in a pot of salted water until tender. Drain well.

7. In a separate pan, heat butter or ghee over medium heat. Add the spinach leaves and sauté until wilted.

8. Mash the cooked sweet potatoes with a potato masher or fork. Add butter or ghee and a splash of milk to achieve a creamy consistency. Season with salt and pepper to taste.

9. Serve the sliced grilled steak alongside a generous portion of sautéed spinach and a dollop of creamy mashed sweet potatoes.

Nutritional Information:

- Calories: 400-450 per serving
- Protein: 30-35g
- Carbohydrates: 30-35g
- Fat: 15-20g
- Fiber: 5-7g

Roasted Chicken Thighs with Roasted Butternut Squash

and Green Beans

Description: Enjoy a comforting and delicious meal featuring succulent roasted chicken thighs, caramelized roasted butternut squash, and vibrant green beans. The roasted chicken thighs are tender and flavorful, while the roasted butternut squash offers a touch of natural sweetness. Paired with crisp green beans, this dish provides a delightful combination of textures and flavors.

Ingredients:

- 4 chicken thighs, bone-in and skin-on
- 1 small butternut squash
- 2 cups fresh green beans
- Olive oil
- Salt and pepper
- Garlic powder
- Paprika
- Dried thyme

Instructions:

1. Preheat the oven to 400°F (200°C).

2. Place the chicken thighs on a baking sheet lined with parchment paper. Drizzle with olive oil and season with salt, pepper, garlic powder, paprika, and dried thyme.

3. Peel and dice the butternut squash into bite-sized

cubes.

4. Toss the butternut squash cubes in a separate bowl with olive oil, salt, and pepper.

5. Spread the seasoned butternut squash cubes on another baking sheet.

6. Place both the chicken thighs and the butternut squash in the preheated oven. Roast for about 25-30 minutes or until the chicken is cooked through and the butternut squash is tender and caramelized.

7. While the chicken and butternut squash are roasting, trim the ends of the green beans.

8. Steam or blanch the green beans until they are tender-crisp.

9. Once the chicken thighs, roasted butternut squash, and green beans are ready, serve them together for a wholesome and satisfying meal.

Nutritional Information:

- Calories: 400-450 per serving
- Protein: 25-30g
- Carbohydrates: 20-25g
- Fat: 20-25g
- Fiber: 5-7g

Turkey Meatballs with Gluten-Free Pasta and Marinara Sauce

Description: Dive into a flavorful and satisfying meal with tender turkey meatballs served over gluten-free pasta and topped with rich marinara sauce. The turkey meatballs are seasoned with herbs and spices, adding a delicious depth of flavor. Paired with gluten-free pasta and tangy marinara sauce, this dish is a comforting and wholesome option that will please everyone at the table.

Ingredients:

- 1 pound ground turkey
- 1/2 cup gluten-free breadcrumbs
- 1/4 cup grated Parmesan cheese
- 1/4 cup chopped fresh parsley
- 1 egg
- 2 cloves garlic, minced
- 1/2 teaspoon dried oregano
- 1/2 teaspoon dried basil
- Salt and pepper
- Gluten-free pasta of your choice
- Marinara sauce (homemade or store-bought)
- Fresh basil leaves for garnish

Instructions:

1. In a large bowl, combine ground turkey, gluten-free breadcrumbs, grated Parmesan cheese, chopped fresh parsley, minced garlic, dried oregano, dried basil, salt, and pepper. Mix until

well combined.

2. Shape the turkey mixture into meatballs of your desired size.

3. Heat olive oil in a large skillet over medium heat. Add the turkey meatballs and cook until browned on all sides and cooked through, about 8-10 minutes.

4. While the meatballs are cooking, prepare the gluten-free pasta according to the package instructions. Drain well.

5. Heat the marinara sauce in a separate saucepan over medium heat until warmed through.

6. Serve the turkey meatballs over a bed of cooked gluten-free pasta. Top with marinara sauce and garnish with fresh basil leaves.

Nutritional Information:

- Calories: 400-450 per serving
- Protein: 25-30g
- Carbohydrates: 30-35g
- Fat: 15-20g
- Fiber: 3-5g

Seared Tuna Steak with Stir-Fried Bok Choy and Jasmine Rice

Description: Indulge in a flavorful and healthy meal featuring seared tuna steak, stir-fried bok choy, and fragrant jasmine rice. The seared tuna steak is tender and succulent, complemented by the crisp and vibrant bok choy. Served alongside fluffy jasmine rice, this dish offers a delightful combination of textures and tastes that will leave you satisfied and nourished.

Ingredients:

- 2 tuna steaks
- 2 baby bok choy
- 2 cups cooked jasmine rice
- Soy sauce
- Sesame oil
- Garlic, minced
- Ginger, grated
- Red pepper flakes (optional)
- Salt and pepper

Instructions:

1. Pat dry the tuna steaks with paper towels. Season with salt, pepper, and a sprinkle of red pepper flakes (if desired).

2. Heat a drizzle of sesame oil in a skillet or grill pan over medium-high heat.

3. Sear the tuna steaks for about 1-2 minutes per side, or until they reach your preferred level of doneness. Remove from the heat and set aside.

4. Cut the bok choy into bite-sized pieces, separating the leaves from the stalks.

5. In the same pan used for the tuna, add a little

more sesame oil if needed. Stir-fry the bok choy stalks, minced garlic, and grated ginger until the stalks are slightly tender.

6. Add the bok choy leaves and continue stir-frying until wilted.

7. Season the stir-fried bok choy with soy sauce to taste.

8. Serve the seared tuna steak alongside the stir-fried bok choy and a side of cooked jasmine rice.

Nutritional Information:

- Calories: 400-450 per serving
- Protein: 30-35g
- Carbohydrates: 30-35g
- Fat: 10-15g
- Fiber: 3-5g

Grilled Pork Tenderloin with Roasted Brussels Sprouts and Wild Rice

Description: Indulge in a hearty and flavorful meal with tender grilled pork tenderloin, roasted Brussels sprouts, and nutty wild rice. The pork tenderloin is marinated and grilled to perfection, while the roasted Brussels sprouts add a delicious caramelized flavor. Paired with wholesome wild rice, this dish offers a delightful combination of textures and tastes that will satisfy your cravings.

Ingredients:

- 1 pork tenderloin
- 1 pound Brussels sprouts
- 1 cup wild rice
- Olive oil
- Dijon mustard
- Maple syrup
- Garlic powder
- Salt and pepper

Instructions:

1. Preheat the grill to medium-high heat.

2. In a small bowl, whisk together olive oil, Dijon mustard, maple syrup, garlic powder, salt, and pepper to create a marinade for the pork tenderloin.

3. Place the pork tenderloin in a shallow dish and pour the marinade over it. Let it marinate for at least 30 minutes, or refrigerate overnight for better flavor.

4. While the pork is marinating, preheat the oven to 400°F (200°C).

5. Trim the Brussels sprouts and cut them in half. Toss them with olive oil, salt, and pepper on a baking sheet.

6. Roast the Brussels sprouts in the preheated oven for about 20-25 minutes, or until they are tender and caramelized.

7. While the Brussels sprouts are roasting, cook the

wild rice according to package instructions. Drain any excess liquid.

8. Grill the marinated pork tenderloin for about 12-15 minutes, turning occasionally, or until the internal temperature reaches 145°F (63°C) for medium doneness.

9. Let the pork tenderloin rest for a few minutes before slicing it into medallions.

10. Serve the grilled pork tenderloin alongside the roasted Brussels sprouts and a portion of cooked wild rice.

Nutritional Information:

- Calories: 400-450 per serving
- Protein: 30-35g
- Carbohydrates: 35-40g
- Fat: 15-20g
- Fiber: 5-7g

Vegetable Curry with Chickpeas and Basmati Rice

Description: Treat yourself to a flavorful and comforting vegetable curry packed with vibrant vegetables, protein-rich chickpeas, and aromatic spices. Served over fragrant basmati rice, this curry is a wholesome and satisfying option for vegetarians and vegans alike. The combination of spices and textures creates a delightful dish that will warm your soul.

Ingredients:

- 1 tablespoon vegetable oil
- 1 onion, diced
- 2 cloves garlic, minced
- 1 tablespoon curry powder
- 1 teaspoon ground cumin
- 1 teaspoon ground coriander
- 1/2 teaspoon turmeric
- 1 can (14 oz) diced tomatoes
- 1 can (14 oz) coconut milk
- 1 cup vegetable broth
- 2 cups mixed vegetables of your choice (such as cauliflower, carrots, bell peppers, peas)
- 1 can (14 oz) chickpeas, drained and rinsed
- Salt and pepper
- Fresh cilantro leaves for garnish
- Cooked basmati rice for serving

Instructions:

1. Heat vegetable oil in a large pot or skillet over medium heat.

2. Add the diced onion and minced garlic to the pot and sauté until the onion is translucent and fragrant.

3. Stir in the curry powder, ground cumin, ground coriander, and turmeric. Cook for an additional minute to toast the spices.

4. Add the diced tomatoes (with their juices),

coconut milk, and vegetable broth to the pot. Stir to combine.

5. Bring the mixture to a simmer and let it cook for about 5 minutes to allow the flavors to meld together.

6. Add the mixed vegetables and chickpeas to the pot. Season with salt and pepper to taste.

7. Cover the pot and let the curry simmer for 15-20 minutes, or until the vegetables are tender.

8. While the curry is simmering, cook the basmati rice according to package instructions.

9. Serve the vegetable curry over a bed of cooked basmati rice. Garnish with fresh cilantro leaves.

Nutritional Information:

- Calories: 350-400 per serving
- Protein: 10-15g
- Carbohydrates: 40-45g
- Fat: 15-20g
- Fiber: 8-10g

Baked Cod with Roasted Asparagus and Quinoa

Description: Enjoy a light and flavorful meal with baked cod, roasted asparagus, and nutty quinoa. The cod fillets are tender and flaky, seasoned with herbs and spices. Paired with roasted asparagus and fluffy quinoa, this dish offers a delightful combination of textures and flavors that will leave you satisfied and nourished.

Ingredients:

- 2 cod fillets
- 1 bunch asparagus
- 1 cup quinoa
- Olive oil
- Lemon juice
- Garlic powder
- Dried dill
- Salt and pepper

Instructions:

1. Preheat the oven to 400°F (200°C).

2. Place the cod fillets on a baking sheet lined with parchment paper. Drizzle with olive oil and season with lemon juice, garlic powder, dried dill, salt, and pepper.

3. Trim the ends of the asparagus spears and arrange them on another baking sheet. Drizzle with olive oil and season with salt and pepper.

4. Bake the cod and asparagus in the preheated oven for about 12-15 minutes, or until the cod is cooked through and flakes easily with a fork, and the asparagus is tender-crisp.

5. While the cod and asparagus are baking, cook the quinoa according to package instructions.

6. Once cooked, fluff the quinoa with a fork and season with salt and pepper to taste.

7. Serve the baked cod on a bed of cooked quinoa, with the roasted asparagus on the side.

Nutritional Information:

- Calories: 300-350 per serving
- Protein: 25-30g
- Carbohydrates: 30-35g
- Fat: 5-8g
- Fiber: 5-7g

Teriyaki Glazed Tofu with Stir-Fried Mixed Vegetables and Brown Rice

Description: Delight in a flavorful and satisfying meal featuring teriyaki-glazed tofu, a colorful stir-fry of mixed vegetables, and nutty brown rice. The tofu is marinated in a tangy teriyaki sauce, creating a savory and sweet glaze. Served alongside a medley of stir-fried vegetables and wholesome brown rice, this dish offers a delightful combination of textures and tastes.

Ingredients:

- 1 block of firm tofu
- 2 cups mixed vegetables (such as bell peppers, broccoli, carrots, snap peas)
- 1 cup cooked brown rice
- Teriyaki sauce (store-bought or homemade)
- Soy sauce

- Sesame oil
- Garlic, minced
- Ginger, grated
- Red pepper flakes (optional)
- Salt and pepper

Instructions:

1. Drain and press the tofu to remove excess moisture. Cut the tofu into cubes.

2. In a bowl, combine teriyaki sauce, soy sauce, sesame oil, minced garlic, grated ginger, red pepper flakes (if desired), salt, and pepper. Stir well to create a marinade.

3. Place the tofu cubes in the marinade and let them soak for at least 30 minutes.

4. Heat a drizzle of sesame oil in a large skillet or wok over medium-high heat.

5. Remove the tofu cubes from the marinade, reserving the marinade for later use.

6. Add the tofu to the skillet and stir-fry until lightly browned on all sides. Remove from the skillet and set aside.

7. In the same skillet, add a little more sesame oil if needed. Stir-fry the mixed vegetables until they are tender-crisp.

8. Pour the reserved marinade over the vegetables and cook for an additional minute to heat through.

9. Serve the teriyaki-glazed tofu alongside the stir-fried mixed vegetables and a portion of cooked

brown rice.

Nutritional Information:

- Calories: 400-450 per serving
- Protein: 15-20g
- Carbohydrates: 50-55g
- Fat: 15-20g
- Fiber: 7-9g

Lemon Herb Roasted Chicken with Roasted Sweet Potatoes and Green Salad

Description: Indulge in a flavorful and comforting meal with lemon herb roasted chicken, roasted sweet potatoes, and a refreshing green salad. The roasted chicken is infused with the bright flavors of lemon and herbs, resulting in juicy and tender meat. Paired with caramelized roasted sweet potatoes and a crisp green salad, this dish offers a delightful combination of flavors and textures.

Ingredients:

- 4 chicken thighs, bone-in and skin-on
- 2 large sweet potatoes
- Mixed salad greens
- Cherry tomatoes
- Cucumber

- Red onion
- Lemon zest
- Fresh herbs (such as rosemary, thyme, or parsley)
- Olive oil
- Garlic powder
- Salt and pepper

Instructions:

1. Preheat the oven to 400°F (200°C).

2. Place the chicken thighs on a baking sheet lined with parchment paper. Drizzle with olive oil and season with lemon zest, minced fresh herbs, garlic powder, salt, and pepper.

3. Peel and chop the sweet potatoes into bite-sized cubes.

4. Toss the sweet potato cubes in a separate bowl with olive oil, salt, and pepper.

5. Spread the seasoned sweet potato cubes on another baking sheet.

6. Roast the chicken thighs and sweet potatoes in the preheated oven for about 25-30 minutes, or until the chicken is cooked through and the sweet potatoes are tender and caramelized.

7. While the chicken and sweet potatoes are roasting, prepare the green salad. In a large bowl, combine mixed salad greens, halved cherry tomatoes, sliced cucumber, and thinly sliced red onion.

8. Drizzle the salad with olive oil and lemon juice. Season with salt and pepper to taste. Toss gently

to combine all the ingredients.

9. Once the chicken thighs, roasted sweet potatoes, and green salad are ready, serve them together for a wholesome and satisfying meal.

Nutritional Information:

- Calories: 400-450 per serving
- Protein: 25-30g
- Carbohydrates: 30-35g
- Fat: 15-20g
- Fiber: 5-7g

Spaghetti Squash with Turkey Bolognese Sauce and a Side of Steamed Broccoli

Description: Enjoy a healthy twist on a classic Italian dish with spaghetti squash topped with flavorful turkey bolognese sauce and a side of steamed broccoli. Spaghetti squash replaces traditional pasta, offering a lighter and lower-carb option. The turkey bolognese sauce is rich and savory, packed with herbs and spices. Paired with steamed broccoli, this dish is both nutritious and delicious.

Ingredients:

- 1 medium spaghetti squash
- 1 pound ground turkey
- 1 can (14 oz) crushed tomatoes
- 1 onion, diced

- 2 cloves garlic, minced
- 1 teaspoon dried basil
- 1 teaspoon dried oregano
- 1/2 teaspoon dried thyme
- Red pepper flakes (optional)
- Olive oil
- Salt and pepper
- Steamed broccoli florets, for serving

Instructions:

1. Preheat the oven to 400°F (200°C).

2. Cut the spaghetti squash in half lengthwise and remove the seeds.

3. Place the spaghetti squash halves on a baking sheet, cut side up. Drizzle with olive oil and season with salt and pepper.

4. Roast the spaghetti squash in the preheated oven for about 40-45 minutes, or until the flesh is tender and easily separates into strands with a fork. Let it cool slightly.

5. While the spaghetti squash is roasting, heat olive oil in a large skillet over medium heat.

6. Add the diced onion and minced garlic to the skillet and sauté until the onion is translucent and fragrant.

7. Add the ground turkey to the skillet and cook until browned and cooked through, breaking it up with a spoon.

8. Stir in the crushed tomatoes, dried basil, dried

oregano, dried thyme, red pepper flakes (if desired), salt, and pepper. Simmer for 10-15 minutes to allow the flavors to meld together.

9. Use a fork to scrape the spaghetti squash flesh into strands. Divide the spaghetti squash strands into serving bowls or plates.

10. Top the spaghetti squash with the turkey bolognese sauce. Serve with steamed broccoli on the side.

Nutritional Information:

- Calories: 350-400 per serving
- Protein: 25-30g
- Carbohydrates: 20-25g
- Fat: 10-15g
- Fiber: 5-7g

Grilled Shrimp with Grilled Zucchini and Quinoa Pilaf

Description: Delight in a light and flavorful meal featuring succulent grilled shrimp, grilled zucchini, and a delightful quinoa pilaf. The grilled shrimp are seasoned to perfection, while the grilled zucchini adds a smoky flavor and tender texture. Served alongside a nutty quinoa pilaf, this dish offers a satisfying combination of flavors and wholesome ingredients.

Ingredients:

- 1 pound shrimp, peeled and deveined

- 2 zucchini
- 1 cup quinoa
- Vegetable or chicken broth
- Olive oil
- Lemon juice
- Garlic powder
- Paprika
- Salt and pepper

Instructions:

1. Preheat the grill to medium-high heat.

2. In a bowl, toss the shrimp with olive oil, lemon juice, garlic powder, paprika, salt, and pepper to coat evenly.

3. Thread the shrimp onto skewers for easier grilling, if desired.

4. Cut the zucchini into slices or halves, lengthwise. Drizzle with olive oil and season with salt and pepper.

5. Grill the shrimp skewers and zucchini slices on the preheated grill for about 2-3 minutes per side, or until the shrimp are pink and cooked through, and the zucchini is tender and slightly charred.

6. While the shrimp and zucchini are grilling, cook the quinoa according to package instructions, substituting vegetable or chicken broth for water to enhance the flavor.

7. Once cooked, fluff the quinoa with a fork and season with salt and pepper to taste.

8. Serve the grilled shrimp and zucchini alongside a portion of quinoa pilaf.

Nutritional Information:

- Calories: 350-400 per serving
- Protein: 25-30g
- Carbohydrates: 30-35g
- Fat: 10-15g
- Fiber: 5-7g

Baked Falafel with a Mediterranean Salad and Gluten-Free Pita Bread

Description: Enjoy a flavorful and satisfying vegetarian meal with baked falafel, a vibrant Mediterranean salad, and gluten-free pita bread. The baked falafel is made from chickpeas and aromatic herbs, providing a delightful texture and taste. Paired with a refreshing Mediterranean salad and gluten-free pita bread, this dish offers a well-rounded and nutritious dining experience.

Ingredients:

- For the falafel:
    - 2 cups cooked chickpeas
    - 1/2 cup chopped fresh parsley
    - 1/2 cup chopped fresh cilantro
    - 1 small onion, chopped
    - 4 cloves garlic, minced

- · 2 tablespoons gluten-free flour (such as chickpea flour)
  - · 1 teaspoon ground cumin
  - · 1 teaspoon ground coriander
  - · 1/2 teaspoon baking powder
  - · Salt and pepper
  - · Olive oil
- · For the Mediterranean salad:
  - · Mixed salad greens
  - · Cherry tomatoes, halved
  - · Cucumber, diced
  - · Red onion, thinly sliced
  - · Kalamata olives
  - · Feta cheese (optional)
  - · Lemon juice
  - · Olive oil
  - · Dried oregano
  - · Salt and pepper
- · Gluten-free pita bread, for serving

Instructions:

1. Preheat the oven to 375°F (190°C).

2. In a food processor, combine the cooked chickpeas, chopped parsley, chopped cilantro, chopped onion, minced garlic, gluten-free flour, ground cumin, ground coriander, baking powder, salt, and pepper. Pulse until the mixture comes together but still has some texture.

3. Shape the falafel mixture into small patties or balls, depending on your preference.

4. Place the falafel patties or balls on a baking sheet lined with parchment paper. Drizzle with olive oil.

5. Bake the falafel in the preheated oven for about 20-25 minutes, or until golden brown and crisp.

6. While the falafel is baking, prepare the Mediterranean salad. In a bowl, combine mixed salad greens, halved cherry tomatoes, diced cucumber, thinly sliced red onion, Kalamata olives, and crumbled feta cheese (if desired).

7. Drizzle the salad with lemon juice, olive oil, dried oregano, salt, and pepper. Toss gently to combine all the ingredients.

8. Warm the gluten-free pita bread according to package instructions.

9. Serve the baked falafel alongside the Mediterranean salad and gluten-free pita bread.

Nutritional Information:

- Calories: 350-400 per serving
- Protein: 10-15g
- Carbohydrates: 40-45g
- Fat: 15-20g
- Fiber: 8-10g

Lemon Garlic Roasted Salmon with Roasted Cauliflower and Quinoa

Description: Indulge in a flavorful and nutritious meal featuring lemon garlic roasted salmon, roasted cauliflower, and quinoa. The salmon fillets are infused with zesty lemon and aromatic garlic, creating a delightful flavor profile. Paired with roasted cauliflower and fluffy quinoa, this dish offers a satisfying combination of textures and tastes that will leave you feeling nourished and satisfied.

Ingredients:

- 2 salmon fillets
- 1 small head of cauliflower
- 1 cup quinoa
- Olive oil
- Lemon juice
- Garlic, minced
- Lemon zest
- Fresh dill (optional)
- Salt and pepper

Instructions:

1. Preheat the oven to 400°F (200°C).

2. Place the salmon fillets on a baking sheet lined with parchment paper. Drizzle with olive oil and season with lemon juice, minced garlic, lemon zest, salt, and pepper.

3. Break the cauliflower into florets and place them on another baking sheet. Drizzle with olive oil and season with salt and pepper.

4. Roast the salmon fillets and cauliflower in the preheated oven for about 12-15 minutes, or until

the salmon is cooked through and flakes easily with a fork, and the cauliflower is tender and caramelized.

5. While the salmon and cauliflower are roasting, cook the quinoa according to package instructions.

6. Once cooked, fluff the quinoa with a fork. Season with salt, pepper, and a drizzle of olive oil to taste.

7. Serve the lemon garlic roasted salmon alongside the roasted cauliflower and a portion of cooked quinoa. Garnish with fresh dill, if desired.

Nutritional Information:

- Calories: 400-450 per serving
- Protein: 25-30g
- Carbohydrates: 30-35g
- Fat: 15-20g
- Fiber: 5-7g

Sautéed Ground Turkey with Mixed Vegetables and Brown Rice Noodles

Description: Enjoy a flavorful and wholesome meal featuring sautéed ground turkey, a medley of mixed vegetables, and brown rice noodles. The ground turkey is cooked with aromatic spices, while the mixed vegetables add color and nutrients to the dish. Paired with gluten-free brown rice noodles, this meal offers a satisfying combination of flavors and textures.

Ingredients:

- 1 pound ground turkey
- 2 cups mixed vegetables (such as bell peppers, carrots, snow peas, mushrooms)
- 8 ounces brown rice noodles
- Soy sauce or tamari (gluten-free soy sauce)
- Sesame oil
- Garlic, minced
- Ginger, grated
- Red pepper flakes (optional)
- Salt and pepper
- Green onions, chopped (for garnish)

Instructions:

1. Cook the brown rice noodles according to package instructions. Drain and set aside.

2. Heat sesame oil in a large skillet or wok over medium heat.

3. Add the minced garlic and grated ginger to the skillet and sauté until fragrant.

4. Add the ground turkey to the skillet and cook until browned and cooked through, breaking it up with a spoon.

5. Stir in the mixed vegetables and cook until they are tender-crisp.

6. Season with soy sauce or tamari, red pepper flakes (if desired), salt, and pepper to taste.

7. Add the cooked brown rice noodles to the skillet and toss to combine all the ingredients.

8. Cook for an additional minute to heat through.

9. Serve the sautéed ground turkey and mixed vegetables with brown rice noodles. Garnish with chopped green onions.

Nutritional Information:

- Calories: 400-450 per serving
- Protein: 25-30g
- Carbohydrates: 40-45g
- Fat: 10-15g
- Fiber: 5-7g

Grilled Vegetable and Halloumi Skewers served with Herbed Quinoa

Description: Enjoy a delightful vegetarian meal with grilled vegetable and halloumi skewers served alongside herbed quinoa. The colorful assortment of grilled vegetables and the deliciously salty halloumi cheese are threaded onto skewers and cooked to perfection. Paired with fragrant herbed quinoa, this dish offers a satisfying combination of flavors and textures that will leave you feeling nourished and satisfied.

Ingredients:

- 1 zucchini
- 1 yellow bell pepper
- 1 red onion
- 8 cherry tomatoes
- 1 block of halloumi cheese
- Olive oil
- Lemon juice
- Fresh herbs (such as basil, parsley, or oregano)
- Salt and pepper
- 1 cup quinoa
- Vegetable broth or water

Instructions:

1. Preheat the grill to medium-high heat.

2. Cut the zucchini, yellow bell pepper, and red onion into chunks or slices, roughly the same size as the cherry tomatoes.

3. Cut the halloumi cheese into cubes.

4. Thread the vegetables and halloumi cubes onto skewers, alternating the ingredients.

5. Drizzle the skewers with olive oil, lemon juice, and sprinkle with salt, pepper, and fresh herbs.

6. Grill the skewers on the preheated grill for about 5-7 minutes per side, or until the vegetables are tender and slightly charred, and the halloumi is golden brown.

7. While the skewers are grilling, rinse the quinoa

under cold water.

8. In a saucepan, bring vegetable broth or water to a boil. Add the rinsed quinoa and cook according to package instructions until the liquid is absorbed and the quinoa is tender.

9. Fluff the cooked quinoa with a fork and add fresh herbs, salt, and pepper to taste.

10. Serve the grilled vegetable and halloumi skewers alongside a portion of herbed quinoa.

Nutritional Information:

- Calories: 350-400 per serving
- Protein: 15-20g
- Carbohydrates: 35-40g
- Fat: 15-20g
- Fiber: 5-7g

Tips for grocery shopping and meal preparation

Grocery shopping and meal preparation play a vital role in successfully following a low FODMAP diet. Here are some helpful tips to make the process easier:

1. **Plan your meals**: Before heading to the grocery store, plan your meals for the week. This will help you create a shopping list and ensure you have all the necessary ingredients.

2. **Read food labels**: When shopping for packaged foods, carefully read the ingredient labels to

check for high FODMAP ingredients such as onion, garlic, high-fructose corn syrup, or certain artificial sweeteners. Look for low FODMAP alternatives or choose fresh, whole foods when possible.

3. **Stick to the perimeter**: In the grocery store, focus on shopping the perimeter where you'll find fresh produce, meat, fish, and dairy alternatives. This will help you avoid the middle aisles that often contain processed foods with hidden FODMAPs.

4. **Stock up on pantry staples**: Keep your pantry stocked with low FODMAP essentials like rice, quinoa, gluten-free oats, canned tomatoes, low FODMAP broths, herbs, and spices. Having these ingredients on hand will make it easier to whip up a low FODMAP meal.

5. **Batch cook and meal prep**: Dedicate some time each week to batch cook and meal prep. Prepare larger quantities of low FODMAP recipes and store them in individual portions for easy grab-and-go meals during busy weekdays.

6. **Freeze leftovers**: If you have leftover meals, consider freezing them in single-serving portions. This will help minimize food waste and provide you with convenient options for future meals.

7. **Experiment with herbs and spices**: While some high FODMAP ingredients like onion and garlic may be off-limits, you can still add flavor to your meals by using herbs and spices that are low FODMAP, such as basil, oregano, ginger, and turmeric.

8. **Keep snacks handy**: Prepare low FODMAP snacks in advance, such as rice cakes, mixed nuts, lactose-free yogurt, or fresh fruit, and keep them easily accessible for when hunger strikes.

9. **Stay hydrated**: Remember to drink plenty of water throughout the day to stay hydrated and support digestion. Herbal teas and infused water can also be enjoyable low FODMAP options.

10. **Seek support**: Consider joining online communities or support groups where you can connect with others following a low FODMAP diet. Sharing experiences, tips, and recipe ideas can be helpful and motivating.

By incorporating these tips into your routine, you'll be better equipped to navigate grocery shopping, meal preparation, and ultimately, maintain a satisfying and nutritious low FODMAP diet.

Remember, it's essential to consult with a healthcare professional or registered dietitian who specializes in digestive health to ensure you're following the low FODMAP diet correctly and meeting your individual nutritional needs.

Chapter five

Reintroducing FODMAPs

Reintroduction Phase and Its Importance

The reintroduction phase is a crucial step in the low FODMAP diet, which is commonly recommended for individuals with irritable bowel syndrome (IBS) or other gastrointestinal issues. FODMAPs, which stands for Fermentable Oligosaccharides, Disaccharides, Monosaccharides, and Polyols, are a group of carbohydrates that can trigger digestive symptoms in sensitive individuals. The initial phase of the low FODMAP diet involves eliminating high FODMAP foods from the diet for a specified period, typically around 2 to 6 weeks. Once the elimination phase is complete and symptoms have improved, the reintroduction phase begins. In this phase, FODMAP-containing foods are gradually reintroduced back into the diet to identify which specific types and amounts of FODMAPs can be tolerated by the individual.

The reintroduction phase is of paramount importance for several reasons. Firstly, it allows individuals to determine their personal tolerance level for different FODMAPs. While some individuals may be highly sensitive to certain types of FODMAPs, others may only experience symptoms with larger quantities. By systematically reintroducing FODMAPs, individuals can identify their specific triggers and create a personalized diet plan that minimizes symptoms while still allowing for dietary variety.

Secondly, the reintroduction phase helps individuals maintain a balanced and sustainable long-term diet. The initial elimination phase can be quite restrictive, as it requires the removal of many commonly consumed foods that are high in FODMAPs. This restriction can lead to nutritional imbalances and potential deficiencies if not carefully managed. The reintroduction phase allows for the reintroduction of a wider range of foods, ensuring that individuals can enjoy a varied and nutritionally adequate diet while still managing their symptoms.

Furthermore, the reintroduction phase provides individuals with a sense of empowerment and control over their diet and symptoms. It allows them to become more attuned to their body's responses to different foods and better understand their unique triggers. Armed with this knowledge, individuals can make informed choices about their dietary intake and confidently navigate social situations that involve food, reducing anxiety and improving overall quality of life.

Guidance on Reintroducing FODMAPs Methodically

When embarking on the reintroduction phase, it is essential to approach it in a methodical and systematic manner. Here is a step-by-step guide to reintroducing FODMAPs:

1. **Choose one FODMAP group at a time:** Start with a single FODMAP group, such as fructose or lactose. This approach allows for a clearer understanding of individual sensitivities and prevents confusion that may arise from reintroducing multiple groups simultaneously.

2. **Start with small amounts:** Begin by consuming a small portion of a food that contains the chosen FODMAP group. It is advisable to start with a low-FODMAP serving size and gradually increase it over a few days, monitoring symptoms along the way.

3. **Monitor symptoms:** Keep a close eye on any changes in symptoms after consuming the reintroduced FODMAP. Symptoms may include bloating, abdominal pain, gas, diarrhea, or constipation. Note down any reactions in a food and symptom diary for reference.

4. **Wait for a few days:** After testing a particular

FODMAP group, return to the low FODMAP diet for a few days, allowing the body to reset and symptoms to settle. This step is crucial for accurately assessing individual tolerances.

5. **Repeat the process for other FODMAP groups:** Once symptoms have settled, move on to reintroducing another FODMAP group using the same method. Proceed gradually, allowing sufficient time to evaluate each group before moving on to the next.

By following this systematic approach, individuals can identify their personal triggers and establish a clear understanding of their tolerance levels for different FODMAPs.

Keeping a Food and Symptom Diary During the Reintroduction Phase

Keeping a food and symptom diary during the reintroduction phase is highly recommended. It serves as a valuable tool for tracking dietary intake and monitoring any associated symptoms. Here are some tips for maintaining an effective food and symptom diary:

1. **Record detailed information:** Include the date, time, and specific foods consumed in your diary. Be as specific as possible, noting portion sizes and preparation methods. This level of detail will help in pinpointing potential triggers.

2. **Track symptoms:** Document any changes or symptoms experienced after consuming reintroduced FODMAPs. Note the severity, duration, and type of symptoms, such as bloating, abdominal pain, or changes in bowel movements. This information will aid in identifying patterns and making connections between specific foods and symptoms.

3. **Consider other factors:** In addition to food intake, record other factors that may impact symptoms, such as stress levels, sleep quality, or medication changes. This broader perspective can provide valuable insights into potential triggers beyond FODMAPs.

4. **Use a rating scale:** Implement a rating scale to assess symptom severity. For example, use a scale from 1 to 10, with 1 indicating minimal symptoms and 10 representing severe symptoms. This will help track symptom progression and identify trends over time.

5. **Review and analyze:** Regularly review your diary to identify patterns or correlations between certain foods and symptoms. Look for consistent reactions or symptom improvements to guide future food choices.

Keeping a food and symptom diary during the reintroduction phase facilitates a systematic and informed approach to identifying personal FODMAP triggers. It empowers individuals to make educated decisions about their diet, promoting symptom management and overall well-being.

CHAPTER FIVE

Managing Challenges and Maintaining the Diet

Coping with Social Situations and Eating Out

Social situations and eating out can present challenges when following a specific diet or dealing with dietary restrictions. However, with some planning and strategies in place, you can navigate these situations more effectively. Here are some tips to help you cope with social situations and eating out while maintaining your dietary needs.

1. **Research the Menu**: Before going to a restaurant or social event, take some time to research the menu. Many restaurants now provide their menus online, allowing you to review the options and identify suitable dishes. Look for items that align with your dietary requirements, such as gluten-free, vegetarian, or low FODMAP options.

2. **Communicate with the Host or Waitstaff**: If you're attending a social gathering or dining at

a restaurant, it's important to communicate your dietary needs to the host or waitstaff. Don't hesitate to ask questions about the ingredients or preparation methods used in the dishes. Most establishments are accommodating and willing to make modifications to accommodate your needs.

3. **Offer to Contribute**: If you're invited to a potluck or gathering, offer to bring a dish that suits your dietary needs. This ensures that you have at least one option available that you can enjoy without any concerns. It also allows you to introduce others to delicious alternatives and raise awareness about your dietary restrictions.

4. **Be Prepared**: If you're unsure about the availability of suitable options, consider eating a small meal or snack before the event. This can help curb hunger and reduce the temptation to indulge in foods that may not align with your dietary requirements. Additionally, you can carry portable snacks or a packed meal to ensure you have something to eat in case the options are limited.

5. **Focus on Socializing**: Remember that social gatherings and eating out are not just about the food. Shift your focus to the company and conversations rather than fixating on what you can or cannot eat. Engage in meaningful conversations, enjoy the atmosphere, and participate in activities to fully embrace the social aspect of the occasion.

6. **Modify Your Order**: Don't be afraid to modify

your order to suit your needs. Ask for substitutions or alterations to make the dish more compatible with your dietary requirements. Most restaurants are willing to accommodate special requests, such as replacing a sauce or dressing, omitting certain ingredients, or adjusting the cooking method.

7. **Bring Your Own Condiments**: If you're following a specific diet, such as a low FODMAP diet, it can be challenging to find suitable condiments or dressings at restaurants. Consider carrying small containers of your favorite low FODMAP condiments, such as salad dressing or sauces, to enhance the flavor of your meal.

8. **Choose Restaurants with Dietary Options**: Seek out restaurants that are known for offering a variety of dietary options. Look for establishments that specialize in gluten-free, vegan, or other specific diets. These restaurants are more likely to have a better understanding of dietary restrictions and offer suitable choices.

9. **Practice Mindful Eating**: When dining out or attending social events, practice mindful eating. Pay attention to your body's hunger and fullness cues, and eat slowly to savor the flavors. This can help you avoid overeating or giving in to cravings that may not align with your dietary needs.

10. **Have a Support System**: Surround yourself with a supportive network of friends, family, or fellow individuals who understand your dietary needs. They can offer encouragement, provide recommendations for suitable restaurants or

recipes, and help you navigate social situations more comfortably.

Remember, it's essential to prioritize your health and dietary needs while still enjoying social situations and eating out. With a little preparation, communication, and mindfulness, you can successfully navigate these scenarios and make choices that align with your well-being.

Dealing with Cravings and Finding Suitable Alternatives

Cravings for certain foods can be challenging, especially when you have dietary restrictions or are trying to follow a specific diet plan. However, there are several strategies you can employ to deal with cravings and find suitable alternatives. Here are some tips to help you navigate cravings while staying on track with your dietary goals.

1. **Identify the Underlying Cause**: Cravings can sometimes be triggered by emotional factors or specific situations. Take a moment to reflect on the possible reasons behind your cravings. Are you experiencing stress, boredom, or emotional distress? Understanding the underlying cause can help you address the root issue and find healthier ways to cope.

2. **Find Substitutes**: Instead of giving in to your cravings for unhealthy foods, look for suitable alternatives that align with your dietary

requirements. For example, if you're craving something sweet, consider having a piece of fruit or a naturally sweetened treat. If you're craving something savory, opt for healthier options like roasted chickpeas or air-popped popcorn.

3. **Plan Your Meals**: Having a well-balanced and satisfying meal plan can help reduce the likelihood of cravings. Ensure that your meals contain a good balance of macronutrients (protein, carbohydrates, and healthy fats) to keep you satiated. Incorporate a variety of flavors and textures to make your meals enjoyable.

4. **Stay Hydrated**: Dehydration can sometimes be mistaken for hunger or cravings. Ensure you're drinking enough water throughout the day to stay properly hydrated. When a craving strikes, try having a glass of water first and see if it subsides.

5. **Distract Yourself**: When a craving arises, distract yourself with a different activity. Engage in a hobby, go for a walk, listen to music, or call a friend. By shifting your attention away from the craving, you can help reduce its intensity and duration.

6. **Practice Mindful Eating**: When you do indulge in your cravings, practice mindful eating. Slow down, savor each bite, and pay attention to the flavors, textures, and sensations. This can enhance your enjoyment and satisfaction, allowing you to be more mindful of portion sizes and make conscious choices.

7. **Seek Support**: Share your cravings and

struggles with a supportive friend, family member, or online community. They can offer encouragement, share their experiences, and provide suggestions for healthier alternatives. Having someone to hold you accountable and cheer you on can make a significant difference in managing cravings.

8. **Address Nutrient Deficiencies**: Sometimes, cravings can be a result of nutrient deficiencies. Ensure that you're meeting your nutritional needs through a well-balanced diet or consider consulting a healthcare professional or registered dietitian to identify any deficiencies and develop a suitable plan.

Remember that occasional indulgence is perfectly fine as long as it's done in moderation and within the limits of your dietary requirements. It's about finding a balance that works for you and making conscious choices that support your overall well-being.

Long-Term Strategies for Incorporating the Low FODMAP Diet into Everyday Life

The low FODMAP diet is an effective approach for managing symptoms of irritable bowel syndrome (IBS) and other digestive disorders. However, incorporating this diet into everyday life may require some adjustments and long-term strategies. Here are some tips to help you successfully integrate the low FODMAP diet into your daily routine.

1. **Educate Yourself**: Take the time to educate yourself about the low FODMAP diet. Understand which foods are high in FODMAPs and which ones are safe to consume in specific quantities. Familiarize yourself with ingredient labels and learn to identify hidden sources of FODMAPs in packaged foods.

2. **Meal Planning**: Plan your meals in advance to ensure you have a variety of low FODMAP options available throughout the week. Look for recipes that are specifically designed for the low FODMAP diet or learn to modify your favorite dishes to make them FODMAP-friendly. This will help you avoid feeling overwhelmed or deprived when it comes to mealtime.

3. **Stock Your Pantry**: Keep your pantry stocked with low FODMAP staples. This includes items like gluten-free flours, canned or dried proteins (such as canned tuna or quinoa), low FODMAP condiments and sauces, and snacks that adhere to the diet. Having these items on hand will make it easier to prepare meals and snacks that fit within the low FODMAP guidelines.

4. **Experiment with Substitutes**: Explore alternative ingredients and substitutes for high FODMAP foods. For example, use lactose-free milk instead of regular milk, replace garlic and onion with garlic-infused oil or the green parts of spring onions, and use gluten-free grains like rice or quinoa instead of wheat-based products. There

are many resources and recipe blogs available that offer creative and delicious low FODMAP alternatives.

5. **Keep a Food Diary**: Keep a food diary to track your symptoms and identify any trigger foods that may be causing issues. This can help you pinpoint specific FODMAPs that may be problematic for you individually. It's also a helpful tool to share with a healthcare professional or registered dietitian, who can provide guidance and support.

6. **Practice Portion Control**: While certain foods may be low FODMAP, consuming large portions of them can still cause symptoms. Be mindful of portion sizes and pay attention to how your body responds to different quantities of FODMAPs. Experiment with portion sizes to find what works best for you.

7. **Be Prepared for Social Situations**: Coping with social situations and eating out while on the low FODMAP diet can be challenging. Prepare ahead by researching restaurants that offer low FODMAP options or by bringing your own meal or snacks if needed. Communicate your dietary needs to others and don't be afraid to ask questions or make special requests.

8. **Seek Support**: Consider joining a support group or connecting with others who are following the low FODMAP diet. Sharing experiences, recipe ideas, and tips with like-minded individuals can make the journey more manageable and enjoyable. Additionally, a registered dietitian with expertise in the low FODMAP diet can provide personalized

guidance and support.

9. **Focus on Overall Gut Health**: While the low FODMAP diet can provide relief from symptoms, it's important to also focus on overall gut health. Incorporate other lifestyle factors that promote gut health, such as regular exercise, stress management techniques, and adequate sleep. A healthy gut can better tolerate FODMAPs and may reduce symptoms over time.

10. **Reintroduce FODMAPs**: After following the low FODMAP elimination phase, work with a healthcare professional or registered dietitian to reintroduce FODMAPs systematically. This will help identify your personal tolerance levels and allow you to expand your diet while still managing symptoms.

Remember that the low FODMAP diet is not meant to be followed indefinitely. It is a temporary elimination diet designed to identify trigger foods and manage symptoms. Working with a healthcare professional or registered dietitian will ensure you receive personalized guidance and support throughout your low FODMAP journey.

Incorporating the low FODMAP diet into everyday life may require some adjustments and planning, but with time and practice, it can become a seamless part of your routine. Stay focused, be patient with yourself, and celebrate the progress you make towards improving your digestive health.

CONCLUSION

Coping with Social Situations and Eating Out

Social situations and eating out can present challenges when following a specific diet or dealing with dietary restrictions. However, with some planning and strategies in place, you can navigate these situations more effectively. Here are some tips to help you cope with social situations and eating out while maintaining your dietary needs.

1. **Research the Menu**: Before going to a restaurant or social event, take some time to research the menu. Many restaurants now provide their menus online, allowing you to review the options and identify suitable dishes. Look for items that align with your dietary requirements, such as gluten-free, vegetarian, or low FODMAP options.

2. **Communicate with the Host or Waitstaff**: If you're attending a social gathering or dining at a restaurant, it's important to communicate your dietary needs to the host or waitstaff. Don't

hesitate to ask questions about the ingredients or preparation methods used in the dishes. Most establishments are accommodating and willing to make modifications to accommodate your needs.

3. **Offer to Contribute**: If you're invited to a potluck or gathering, offer to bring a dish that suits your dietary needs. This ensures that you have at least one option available that you can enjoy without any concerns. It also allows you to introduce others to delicious alternatives and raise awareness about your dietary restrictions.

4. **Be Prepared**: If you're unsure about the availability of suitable options, consider eating a small meal or snack before the event. This can help curb hunger and reduce the temptation to indulge in foods that may not align with your dietary requirements. Additionally, you can carry portable snacks or a packed meal to ensure you have something to eat in case the options are limited.

5. **Focus on Socializing**: Remember that social gatherings and eating out are not just about the food. Shift your focus to the company and conversations rather than fixating on what you can or cannot eat. Engage in meaningful conversations, enjoy the atmosphere, and participate in activities to fully embrace the social aspect of the occasion.

6. **Modify Your Order**: Don't be afraid to modify your order to suit your needs. Ask for substitutions or alterations to make the dish more

compatible with your dietary requirements. Most restaurants are willing to accommodate special requests, such as replacing a sauce or dressing, omitting certain ingredients, or adjusting the cooking method.

7. **Bring Your Own Condiments**: If you're following a specific diet, such as a low FODMAP diet, it can be challenging to find suitable condiments or dressings at restaurants. Consider carrying small containers of your favorite low FODMAP condiments, such as salad dressing or sauces, to enhance the flavor of your meal.

8. **Choose Restaurants with Dietary Options**: Seek out restaurants that are known for offering a variety of dietary options. Look for establishments that specialize in gluten-free, vegan, or other specific diets. These restaurants are more likely to have a better understanding of dietary restrictions and offer suitable choices.

9. **Practice Mindful Eating**: When dining out or attending social events, practice mindful eating. Pay attention to your body's hunger and fullness cues, and eat slowly to savor the flavors. This can help you avoid overeating or giving in to cravings that may not align with your dietary needs.

10. **Have a Support System**: Surround yourself with a supportive network of friends, family, or fellow individuals who understand your dietary needs. They can offer encouragement, provide recommendations for suitable restaurants or recipes, and help you navigate social situations more comfortably.

Remember, it's essential to prioritize your health and dietary needs while still enjoying social situations and eating out. With a little preparation, communication, and mindfulness, you can successfully navigate these scenarios and make choices that align with your well-being.

Dealing with Cravings and Finding Suitable Alternatives

Cravings for certain foods can be challenging, especially when you have dietary restrictions or are trying to follow a specific diet plan. However, there are several strategies you can employ to deal with cravings and find suitable alternatives. Here are some tips to help you navigate cravings while staying on track with your dietary goals.

1. **Identify the Underlying Cause**: Cravings can sometimes be triggered by emotional factors or specific situations. Take a moment to reflect on the possible reasons behind your cravings. Are you experiencing stress, boredom, or emotional distress? Understanding the underlying cause can help you address the root issue and find healthier ways to cope.

2. **Find Substitutes**: Instead of giving in to your cravings for unhealthy foods, look for suitable alternatives that align with your dietary requirements. For example, if you're craving something sweet, consider having a piece of fruit or a naturally sweetened treat. If you're craving

something savory, opt for healthier options like roasted chickpeas or air-popped popcorn.

3. **Plan Your Meals**: Having a well-balanced and satisfying meal plan can help reduce the likelihood of cravings. Ensure that your meals contain a good balance of macronutrients (protein, carbohydrates, and healthy fats) to keep you satiated. Incorporate a variety of flavors and textures to make your meals enjoyable.

4. **Stay Hydrated**: Dehydration can sometimes be mistaken for hunger or cravings. Ensure you're drinking enough water throughout the day to stay properly hydrated. When a craving strikes, try having a glass of water first and see if it subsides.

5. **Distract Yourself**: When a craving arises, distract yourself with a different activity. Engage in a hobby, go for a walk, listen to music, or call a friend. By shifting your attention away from the craving, you can help reduce its intensity and duration.

6. **Practice Mindful Eating**: When you do indulge in your cravings, practice mindful eating. Slow down, savor each bite, and pay attention to the flavors, textures, and sensations. This can enhance your enjoyment and satisfaction, allowing you to be more mindful of portion sizes and make conscious choices.

7. **Seek Support**: Share your cravings and struggles with a supportive friend, family member, or online community. They can offer encouragement, share their experiences, and

provide suggestions for healthier alternatives. Having someone to hold you accountable and cheer you on can make a significant difference in managing cravings.

8. **Address Nutrient Deficiencies**: Sometimes, cravings can be a result of nutrient deficiencies. Ensure that you're meeting your nutritional needs through a well-balanced diet or consider consulting a healthcare professional or registered dietitian to identify any deficiencies and develop a suitable plan.

Remember that occasional indulgence is perfectly fine as long as it's done in moderation and within the limits of your dietary requirements. It's about finding a balance that works for you and making conscious choices that support your overall well-being.

Long-Term Strategies for Incorporating the Low FODMAP Diet into Everyday Life

The low FODMAP diet is an effective approach for managing symptoms of irritable bowel syndrome (IBS) and other digestive disorders. However, incorporating this diet into everyday life may require some adjustments and long-term strategies. Here are some tips to help you successfully integrate the low FODMAP diet into your daily routine.

1. **Educate Yourself**: Take the time to educate

yourself about the low FODMAP diet. Understand which foods are high in FODMAPs and which ones are safe to consume in specific quantities. Familiarize yourself with ingredient labels and learn to identify hidden sources of FODMAPs in packaged foods.

2. **Meal Planning**: Plan your meals in advance to ensure you have a variety of low FODMAP options available throughout the week. Look for recipes that are specifically designed for the low FODMAP diet or learn to modify your favorite dishes to make them FODMAP-friendly. This will help you avoid feeling overwhelmed or deprived when it comes to mealtime.

3. **Stock Your Pantry**: Keep your pantry stocked with low FODMAP staples. This includes items like gluten-free flours, canned or dried proteins (such as canned tuna or quinoa), low FODMAP condiments and sauces, and snacks that adhere to the diet. Having these items on hand will make it easier to prepare meals and snacks that fit within the low FODMAP guidelines.

4. **Experiment with Substitutes**: Explore alternative ingredients and substitutes for high FODMAP foods. For example, use lactose-free milk instead of regular milk, replace garlic and onion with garlic-infused oil or the green parts of spring onions, and use gluten-free grains like rice or quinoa instead of wheat-based products. There are many resources and recipe blogs available that offer creative and delicious low FODMAP alternatives.

5. **Keep a Food Diary**: Keep a food diary to track your symptoms and identify any trigger foods that may be causing issues. This can help you pinpoint specific FODMAPs that may be problematic for you individually. It's also a helpful tool to share with a healthcare professional or registered dietitian, who can provide guidance and support.

6. **Practice Portion Control**: While certain foods may be low FODMAP, consuming large portions of them can still cause symptoms. Be mindful of portion sizes and pay attention to how your body responds to different quantities of FODMAPs. Experiment with portion sizes to find what works best for you.

7. **Be Prepared for Social Situations**: Coping with social situations and eating out while on the low FODMAP diet can be challenging. Prepare ahead by researching restaurants that offer low FODMAP options or by bringing your own meal or snacks if needed. Communicate your dietary needs to others and don't be afraid to ask questions or make special requests.

8. **Seek Support**: Consider joining a support group or connecting with others who are following the low FODMAP diet. Sharing experiences, recipe ideas, and tips with like-minded individuals can make the journey more manageable and enjoyable. Additionally, a registered dietitian with expertise in the low FODMAP diet can provide personalized guidance and support.

9. **Focus on Overall Gut Health**: While the low FODMAP diet can provide relief from symptoms,

it's important to also focus on overall gut health. Incorporate other lifestyle factors that promote gut health, such as regular exercise, stress management techniques, and adequate sleep. A healthy gut can better tolerate FODMAPs and may reduce symptoms over time.

10. **Reintroduce FODMAPs**: After following the low FODMAP elimination phase, work with a healthcare professional or registered dietitian to reintroduce FODMAPs systematically. This will help identify your personal tolerance levels and allow you to expand your diet while still managing symptoms.

Remember that the low FODMAP diet is not meant to be followed indefinitely. It is a temporary elimination diet designed to identify trigger foods and manage symptoms. Working with a healthcare professional or registered dietitian will ensure you receive personalized guidance and support throughout your low FODMAP journey.

Incorporating the low FODMAP diet into everyday life may require some adjustments and planning, but with time and practice, it can become a seamless part of your routine. Stay focused, be patient with yourself, and celebrate the progress you make towards improving your digestive health.